COOLING FOR LYMPHEDEMA

ADVANCES IN TREATING LYMPHEDEMA

Jean A. Yzer P.T.

South Florida Breast Cancer Rehab Center

275 NW 107th Ave

Pembroke Pines, FL 33026

www.soflbreastrehab.org

JeanYzer@soflbreastrehab.org

Book Layout ©2017 BookDesignTemplates.com

Book Cover Art by Michael Colanero www.uncommonstock.net. **The Breast Cancer Awareness Body Painting Project – A Fine Art & Photography Essay of Survivors**. Raising awareness, offering hope and inspiration worldwide. Image on last page "Warrior" body painting of Maria Santaella.

Cooling for Lymphedema: Advances in Treating Lymphedema / Jean A. Yzer -- 1st ed.

ISBN: 154649829X
ISBN-13: 978-1546498292

To all persons living with lymphedema,
may your path be lighter.

Acknowledgements

This book would not have been possible without the many people who crossed my path. From my early teachers, including my parents Rudi and Isabella who taught me to believe in myself, to all my patients who trusted my direction. In particular Dr. Elizabeth Tan Chiu, who opened the door to this discovery, and Dr. Harvey Mayrovitz whose expertise was the bridge to validate this treatment.

Contents

Introduction

I have lost track how many of my patients over the years have said to me, "I went through cancer and chemotherapy and now this?" *This* meaning lymphedema. Secondary lymphedema to be exact, the kind that results after trauma *or* cancer surgery, when lymph nodes and lymphatic tissue are removed. It seems unfair, outrageous actually. And then to be told that lymphedema could not be cured and was a progressive disease?

Even to me, burdened by intricate knowledge about the lymphatic system, this did not really make sense. Why should secondary lymphedema be a logical consequence of cancer-related surgery in which lymphatic tissue is harvested to reduce the risk of cancer cells spreading? Rehabilitation specialists are faced with swelling all the time. Why is this swelling so vastly different that we cannot do a better job at minimizing the risk factors and consequences? From the first time I heard the theory of a correlation of necessity between lymphedema and the surgical knife into lymphatic tissue, I was skeptical. Something was not stacking up. So I took it upon myself to investigate the knowledge base further in search of answers.

I am glad I did not take a back seat to standard views! What I have discovered about lymphedema, first by clinical experimentation and then by scientific inquiry, is already changing lives. I might not have undertaken this journey if not for the inspiration from my patients to think out of the box and explore an unrecognized, simple, and now proven treatment method to make you better prepared to manage lymphedema. If you, my reader, are a patient, or if you are so lucky to be a health professional who is called upon to assist others in managing their lymphedema, here you will find knowledge that will help you. The cooling method for lymphedema you will read about was originally created on patients with secondary lymphedema. My clinical experience has since shown that not just secondary lymphedema from cancer related surgical procedures and treatments, but other forms of lymphedema show favorable responds to topical skin cooling. Scientific research must continue to expand the knowledge base in those areas not yet studied to establish treatment parameters and make this treatment available to all who suffer.

If you have chronic lymphedema, you will quickly recognize that I am introducing a treatment called topical skin cooling that you have not yet heard about from your lymphedema therapist. If lymphedema is new to you, let me tell you that though you will be reading about a treatment option with scientific merit, I encourage you to find a lymphedema therapist to guide you on your path. The individuals who have the best results managing their lymphedema have educated themselves on all standard treatment options and have created an individualized treatment plan with the help of a specialist. Topical skin cooling does not stand on its own. It enhances and works best in conjunction with all other standard treatment options currently available.

Finding what works comes by a process of trial and discovery. You must learn to navigate the world of bandaging and compression options. But first of all you must learn what you are dealing with. Knowledge is power, but don't believe everything you are told. As I did, always investigate. At those times that you need support, lean on a trusted health care provider.

But always take back your power when you have regained your strength. And strength, as far as I am concerned, is more of an inner than outer nature. Illness such as cancer can leave you feeling depleted of creative strength but you need not stay there. In a later chapter we will touch on the power of a healing mind-set, one of my favorite subjects, itself worthy of an entire book.

Lymphedema will have you pay attention to it. Learning what it is and what it isn't, will give you confidence to walk your path. What you will find here will empower you to take better command of your lymphedema and therefore your life. What if I told you right now, that lymphedema will not stand in your way of living your dreams!

CHAPTER 1

From a Traditional to a Broader Perspective

The Beginning

Did you ever look back to the time before a change occurred to see if there were any indications you had missed before hand? The day my life as a lymphedema therapist changed appeared to be an ordinary day at the clinic. But there is one thing I *can* say: I had known for some time there was a piece missing to the puzzle of treating lymphedema, especially as it concerned acute lymphedema. I am defining acute swelling as the time that starts right after the swelling begins, when it first appears, sometimes right after surgery, sometimes gradually but distinctly, sometimes rapidly, even overnight, and usually accompanied by heat, pain, stiffness, fear and disbelief.

In my lymphedema clinic located in an oncology office, I was brought face to face on a regular basis with the immediacy and stark reality of acute lymphedema. Oncologists see their patients before and after cancer surgery, and during and after chemotherapy and radiation therapy. Lymphedema can and does appear at all of those times. They see their patients when something all of a sudden goes different than expected. Once a lymphatic obstruction sets in, rapid resolve is key for the tissue to return to its normal state. The longer the tissue remains stretched, the harder it will be to return to what previously was considered a baseline state.

Not a day would go by that the doctor, wouldn't walk into my treatment room to ask if I could help a patient sitting in the evaluation room with swelling, pain or other physical impairment related to surgery or treatment for cancer. More often than not, the pain was due to an acute onset of swelling. I would always say yes, of course I could help, though in the beginning making sure not to show just how unsure I felt about really being able to make a difference and help the patient.

First Attempt at Cooling

On that day a lady was referred to me who had developed painful swelling in her arm and breast. She had been diagnosed with breast cancer and had already undergone chemotherapy, a lumpectomy to remove a tumor in her breast, and was receiving radiation therapy when the swelling suddenly began. She became alarmed at the rapid onset of swelling in her breast and arm and called the doctor. Of course she suspected the worst, that the cancer had returned. Who wouldn't? When I assessed her distended skin I noted that it was warm, firm, and she could barely stand to be touched because of the pain.

Traditional lymphedema management, would have me start a lymphatic drainage massage once the patient was medically cleared for treatment by the doctor. If there is any indication of an acute medical condition, called a cellulitis infection, lymphatic treatment would be contraindicated and held for a very good reason, to prevent a rapid spread of the infection and put the patient's life at risk. In that case medical and pharmaceutical treatment takes precedence. Luckily for me, I had medical clearance since there was no evidence of a cellulitis infection as confirmed by the initial blood test done in the doctor's office, but what I did not have yet was a viable treatment. Compression, another treatment alternative, was also not an option as this patient was in too much discomfort to tolerate firm contact. The patient was on my treatment table and more than anything I wanted to help.

In hindsight, I realized that my training as a physical therapist had prepared me very well for just that occasion. The idea occurred to me to immerse washcloths into a basin of cold water, a mixture of ice cubes and water, and to cool the tender skin by contouring the washcloths to the involved swollen breast and upper arm. Despite the difference in temperature between the cold washcloth and the warm skin, my patient immediately welcomed the change in temperature with a sigh of relief. After repeating this process three or four times, her pain had disappeared, the tissue of the breast and upper arm had become softer, and the skin temperature was reduced. For those who appreciate pain scales, the patient went from a top level pain rating to the bottom of the scale. The physical agent of cold therapy for reducing swelling and pain trusted by rehabilitation specialists worldwide, had once again worked its magic!

Even though The APTA – American Physical Therapy Association Guide to Physical Therapy practice lists cryotherapy and compression as treatment options for lymphedema, cryotherapy is not commonly utilized in lymphedema care, nor is it instructed as a standard treatment option in the training programs for lymphedema therapists. LANA – The Lymphology

Association of North America in its Position Paper Lymphedema Risk Reduction Practices lists extremes of temperature, both cold and heat, as risk factors for lymphedema. There is a vast range of degrees between extreme cold which presumably means freezing temperatures and moderate cooling, where the temperature stays far above freezing. Freezing temperatures can have long term damaging impact on microvasculature and reduce lymph movement even further. However no study had looked at the therapeutic benefits of topical skin cooling for lymphedema management where the cooling temperatures applied to often delicate human tissue where sensation had been altered by multiple surgical and medical treatments for cancer, were kept in a moderate range to prevent damage and discomfort.

On that day, following the unexpected success of my first attempt at applying topical skin cooling to acute lymphedema of the breast, I offered my patient a short sequence of decongestive massage therapy. She also participated in arm and shoulder stretches and exercises to activate the muscle pumping activity, one of the natural means of moving lymphatic fluid throughout the body. She went home that day with instructions to continue to apply cool washcloths to her breast and arm, and perform her stretches and exercises. A few days later, at the second visit, her swelling was resolved, her functional range of movement was normal, and the patient was happy with her progress. And best of all, her outlook had entirely changed. Gone were all morbid thoughts. She had renewed confidence she would complete her radiation therapy and resume a life of quality. I followed up with her one more time during her radiation therapy treatment and also fitted her with a compression garment.

Eye-Opening Conclusion

This next statement is no rocket science: Textbooks never do the whole story justice. A larger reality becomes evident when one comes face-to-face with the patient living with lymphedema. There is yet another experience that textbooks perhaps *cannot* do justice and therapists rarely see. When the lymphedema is at its most acute, when the patient first gets to the doctor's office, before medical treatment is offered, when the patient is in pain and fear from having witnessed, sometimes overnight, the sudden swelling of an arm or a breast. Not all lymphedema comes on this fast, much of it comes on gradually in the months and years after surgery. Having been at the front line, and witnessed the acute presentation of lymphedema, has given me insight into some of the pieces clinicians might have been missing about treating the set of symptoms we call lymphedema and classify as a disease. Therapists also rarely see the patient right after surgery, when the surgical bandages come off the chest, while the surgical draining tubes are still in. In most cases, the lymphedema therapist sees the patient further down the road, when the swelling has been present for a few weeks, a few months or even years. The fact that many therapists do not see lymphedema in its most acute state may well be the reason why topical skin cooling, the subject of the scientific study I co-authored, and the topic of this book, has not been utilized to date as standard protocol in the treatment of all lymphedema. What else could explain why we are treating lymphedema so differently than other swelling?

Secondary lymphedema is typically caused by an obstruction in the lymphatic vessels caused by trauma or a disease process that results in a back-up and accumulation of protein-rich fluid in the surrounding cellular tissue. Lymphatic fluid is a normally occurring fluid in the body, but the accumulation of this fluid is not a normal condition. The word lymphedema literally breaks down to *edema* or *swelling* which contains *lymph* fluid. Any time there is swelling in the body, lymphatic fluid likely makes up a part of that swelling. Swelling in the human body can technically contain any fluid normally occurring, most often this will be blood and lymphatic fluid. When there is an infection the lymph fluid will contain a buildup of white blood cells and may be referred to as pus.

When it comes to swelling related to trauma such as a sports injury, an accident, or orthopedic surgery, our first instinct is to apply a cool compress. We also commonly apply cooling during the healing process when the swelling lingers. There are well founded concerns regarding applying extreme cold temperatures to human skin as this is known to cause ischemia and permanent damage to microvasculature. In the management of swelling resulting from secondary lymphedema we are treating the superficial lymphatic system, a system located just below the skin. If no medically prohibiting concerns exist, why would we not apply a modified version of a cool compress to secondary lymphedema, be it in an acute presentation, a mild or a chronic case? There is no evidence, nor rational reason to believe, that topical skin cooling when applied in a safe temperature range causes harm to human tissue. And its benefit in the clinical management of lymphedema until now simply had not yet been studied and known. Is there swelling and then another kind of swelling we are calling lymphedema? The answer most commonly given to differentiate the cause of lymphedema from all other swelling is that it is a mechanical insufficiency of the lymphatic system. But mechanical cause is never the sole informer of treatment, and when it comes to applying topical cooling to human skin, we already have a vast database of clinical evidence to lean on. Do you feel, as I did, that there is something missing here?

By working with acute and chronic cases of lymphedema for the past ten years, I learned that the initial treatment for lymphedema should immediately be geared to decreasing the inflammatory process present in the lymphatic system and surrounding tissue. In my clinical experience and subsequent research, I discovered that topical skin cooling swiftly improves the symptoms of inflammation, swelling, tissue firmness, pain, and skin temperature over areas impacted by lymphedema. Because topical skin cooling immediately begins to decrease the inflammation in tissue, it also positively impacts the long term effects of this potentially progressive disorder. What I am suggesting is that how we treat lymphedema when it first arises may well hold the key to reducing the presentation we now know and accept as normal, as chronic lymphedema. This is big. This is life changing for anyone at risk for, and living with lymphedema.

CHAPTER 2

Exploring Lymphedema

What Does the Lymphatic System Do?

Mammals contain two vascular systems: the blood and the lymphatic system. More people these days have heard of the lymphatic system though many are still mystified what this system actually does. The heart pumps blood under pressure throughout the body. The blood exits the bloodstream by leaking out into the interstitium at the capillary beds on its route to deliver nutrients and oxygen to the cells. The cells absorb the needed molecules for metabolism, releasing the by products back to the interstitial space for removal by the lymphatic system.

Under normal circumstances the lymphatic system has two important functions. It is the fluid medium that transports cellular waste away from cells to the periphery of the body where it is excreted, and the lymphatic system is also an integral part of your immune and repair system.

Just as in any form of combustion, once the cells have used the sugars from the foods you eat and oxygen from the air you breath to metabolize the energy your muscles and your brain use, waste products have to be removed. Utilizing a pressure gradient created by solution of molecules into liquid, the lymphatic fluid is the medium by which metabolic waste is removed. An intricate system of lymphatic vessels that originate in smaller diameter vessels and end up as larger ones merge with the venous circulatory system and transports the waste products to our excretory systems. It is important that this transport system functions efficiently since waste products that remain in the tissue create a toxic environment where disease can manifest. Roughly speaking we could say that in this capacity the lymphatic system is the waste removal mechanism of our body that functions as the plumbing and sewer systems do in our homes.

The lymphatic system also plays an important role in the immune defense of our bodies. Within the lymphatic system are the important lymph nodes. The first function of lymph nodes is to filter and cleanse the fluid that flows through the lymphatic vessels. Lymphocytes are the white blood cells responsible for much of the body's immune system. Everyone reading this book will know that white blood cells are the soldiers of the immune system that protect us from disease. These cells that originate in the bone marrow lie in the lymph nodes, the spleen and other lymphoid organs where they have maximum contact with foreign bodies, while a lesser amount circulate in the blood ready to travel anywhere in the body bacteria and toxins are detected. The white blood cells are capable of encasing the invading organisms and breaking them down into smaller component parts for easy removal from the body. You want your immune system to be functioning optimally and the white blood cells to be able to travel unhindered throughout the body. Whenever there is stagnant fluid, such as with lymphedema, white blood cells may not be able to penetrate through a congested area fast enough to prevent invading organisms from multiplying. Additionally, stagnant fluid traps body heat which offers optimal conditions for the growth of organisms. Without white blood cells in place, an infection can develop and spread rapidly.

What is Secondary Lymphedema?

Traditional theory informs us that secondary lymphedema results from mechanical changes brought on by permanent damage from surgical trauma to the lymphatic system. The lymphatic system, which is made up of a vast network of vessels connected by lymph nodes that literally covers and supports your entire body in maintaining health, may also have been permanently altered by the growth of a tumor in or around the lymph nodes and lymphatic vessels.

What a mechanical failure of the lymphatic system means, is that the system is unable to handle the usual amount of lymphatic fluid passing through the area and this results in a back-up and back-flow of fluid. Luckily for us, there is redundancy built into the lymphatic system, allowing fluid to flow through other existing lymphatic pathways and bypass the damaged area. There is a limit to which the lymphatic system can be altered and recover before there is a deterioration of function. A situation of chronic back-flow of fluid causes the characteristic swelling and distention we refer to as secondary lymphedema, that requires daily maintenance to manage.

One of the reasons I limit the discussion to secondary lymphedema is that the scientific study I co-authored titled *Local Skin Cooling as an Aid to the Management of Patients with Breast Cancer Related Lymphedema and Fibrosis of the Arm or*

Breast (Mayrovitz, Yzer, Lymphology 50(2017)56-66), primarily evaluated the utility of cooling in this diagnosis class. Though I have experimented with topical skin cooling treatment for patients with other types of lymphedema, there is as yet no scientific study to back up those clinical findings. Further study is needed to determine the impact of cooling in other presentations of lymphedema and establish safe treatment parameters.

Another medical presentation of secondary lymphedema, which is not the subject of this book, is related to progressive heart failure when physical changes in the cardiovascular system result in the pooling of venous blood in the lower extremities. Since the cardiovascular system and the lymphatic system are intricately related, a backup in the venous system will also impact the lymphatic system causing swelling in the legs. We usually associate this process with an aging venous system, as the elderly are more prone to experiencing secondary lymphedema caused by venous insufficiency.

Primary lymphedema, also not the subject of this book, is another type of lymphedema. It is characterized by the incomplete development of the lymphatic system. It is dictated by genetics and results in the lymphatic system being compromised at some point in development. Primary lymphedema may not show up until puberty or even later in life. There are other types of lymphedema found in third world countries which are not discussed in this book.

Common Descriptors of Lymphedema

A common description of secondary lymphedema in the literature is that it is manageable but not curable. Let's have a closer look at this. Not curable, though not technically incorrect when referring to the permanent physical changes that occur in the course of the surgical and medical treatments for cancer, may give the expression that lymphedema is not preventable. Not curable also implies that lymphedema could be a disease. We should pause and at least question the current classification of lymphedema as a disease. One does not catch secondary lymphedema, it is not contagious. In this book we will be exploring that secondary lymphedema appears to originate as an effect, which then becomes cause to a chain reaction of breakdowns resulting in chronic swelling, tissue fibrosis, infections, disfigurement of the affected body part, and decreased function and quality of life.

Mechanical Process, Inflammatory Process, or Both

The fact that long-term effects of low-level inflammation can have a progressive and destructive impact on the lymphatic system has already been written about (Zuther J, Lymphedema Management). It would appear however, that the rationale of lymphedema as a progressive inflammatory process has not found its way with sufficient impact into the available treatment options for this condition. The inflammatory process inherent in lymphedema is currently not managed by treatment options commonly used in the management of inflammatory conditions such as pharmaceuticals or traditional physical modalities, as the topical skin cooling discussed here. Clinicians have not understood why lymphedema occurred in one person but not in another. Why it manifests immediately after surgery in some patients but shows up only years later in others. Why some people living with lymphedema have more frequent episodes of cellulitis infections than others. What have we been missing in our understanding of why lymphedema develops and progresses?

The lymphatic vessel is commonly understood to be a string of lymphangions where lymph is collected and travels on its journey back to the venous circulation. Along the way the lymph fluid also passes through lymph nodes where it is filtered. The textbook explanation for the progressive destruction of the lymphatic system that leads to chronic swelling focuses on the impact of the gradual loss of functional integrity of the lymphangion, the unit of the lymph vessel in between two one-way valves. The sequence commonly described is that a back up of fluid leads to distention of the collecting vessels, a subsequent weakening and then overload of the intrinsic lymphatic pump, and finally to complete incompetence of the unit.

Under normal circumstances the smooth musculature in the cell wall lining of the lymphangion responds to reaching a maximum level of fill by an involuntary contraction that propels a bolus of lymph fluid forward, closing the one-way valve behind it to prevent gravitational backflow. When lymph fluid cannot advance, the internal pressure will build, overstretching the smooth musculature and shutting down the natural contractile impulse of the unit. Without this response the lymph vessels are rendered incapable of moving fluid independently, relying instead on the far less effective method of advancing lymph fluid, the pumping action of the surrounding voluntary skeletal muscles. Traditional dogma has it that lymph fluid will be forced backwards through the collecting system into the interstitial space where it pools and alters the pH and health of the tissue. This is also where the coagulation of stagnant protein molecules will result in the formation of fibrotic patches which harden the tissue, further impeding lymph movement. Newer research suggests (Triacca et al, Circulation Research) that lymphatic solute can also be transported transcellular, across the lumen of the lymph vessel, adding to the known ways the lymphatic system can respond when the inner pressure increases. In cases of inflammation when white blood cells are rapidly mobilized, transcellular movement of particles would appear to be an effective transport method.

What the distinction between a mechanical and inflammatory origin to lymphedema means to the reader with an impaired lymphatic system, is that though the mechanical changes resulting from surgery and cancer related treatments cannot easily be repaired, it is conceivable that by paying better attention to and managing the low level inflammatory aspect of lymphedema we will be better able to prevent progressive damage to the lymphatic system. Without which lymphedema does *not* become a chronic condition elevated to the status of a disease, as it currently is defined by The International Statistical Classification of Diseases and Related Health Problems.

There already exists a body of knowledge about the impact of chronic inflammation on human tissue. Low grade chronic inflammation in any system in the human body is known to cause progressive damage that can lead to disease (Osiecki, H, Altern Med Rev). Medical specialists in the field of lymphedema need to start asking new questions. Such as, does the presence of concurring medical diagnoses, known allergies, and immune system dysfunction that predisposes for low grade inflammation increase the risk of an individual developing secondary lymphedema? And how can lingering inflammation affecting the lymphatic system be prevented from escalating before irreparable damage is done to the tissue?

CHAPTER 3

Lymphedema: Cause or Effect

Definition of a Disease

Though lymphedema is classified as a disease and has defining ICD-codes, to the practicing clinician lymphedema might be better defined as a condition. The rehabilitation specialist might also say it has the markers of a disability as it impedes mobility, function and quality of life. We might take pause and ask ourselves why there is confusion in defining what lymphedema actually is.

There are several good definitions of a disease readily available from the National Institute of Health and Merriam-Webster Dictionary. These definitions all identify a disease as a pathological condition that occurs from various causes, impairs normal functioning of body systems and organs, and has distinguishing signs and symptoms. The term "various causes" refers to both external factors such as pathogens that cause infections, genetic defect, environmental stressors, and internal factors which refer to immune system dysfunction. In the human body, the term "disease" is broadly used to refer to conditions that cause pain, disability, distress, or social problems. No lymphedema specialist would argue that fully developed secondary lymphedema has all the markers used to define disease.

Benefits of Classification as a Disease

In the medical field classifying a condition as a disease has many advantages. It is an accepted method of enabling communication between professionals and it also provides a guide for streamlining treatment parameters, for prognosis, and for insurance reimbursement. In addition, it provides a basis for establishing the need for research and facilitates the data collection process. Besides aiding in early diagnosing, which is of foremost importance in preventing the progression of lymphedema, it also facilitates the disbursement of up-to-date clinical treatment information.

From Effect to Cause

To the closely observing eye, in the process of lymphedema becoming fully expressed, something unusual occurs, effect becomes cause. The effects of the surgical procedure, the early swelling caused by the initial inflammatory response and the physical changes in the lymphatic system result in a chronic condition, that then becomes cause to other medical diagnoses.

When a patient presents to a lymphedema clinic the most frequently seen signs and symptoms are pain, swelling, a history of infections known as cellulitis infections, fibrosis or hardening of tissue, restrictions in joint movement, myofascial or soft tissue restrictions known as Axillary Web Syndrome or cording, and even nerve entrapments. A few well placed questions will also reveal evidence of the less visible human factor, the emotional cost, and the impact on professional, social and family life.

Piercing the Origin of Lymphedema

Lymphedema starts out as a natural healing response by the body. When surgery is performed, *local* swelling or congestion occurs at the site of the surgical incision. Local swelling may be temporary or may linger as residual congestion as seen in slow healing wounds or infections. Any trauma to the body will result in a leakage of fluid from ruptured vasculature, both arterial and venous, as well as lymphatic. This fluid will seep into the surrounding tissue and cause congestion or swelling. When by incision of the surgical knife the network of lymphatic vessels is cut, the healing process of this delicate tissue must involve scarring. The body, in its infinite wisdom, will heal the ruptured area by creating new connecting tissue, new collagen fibers. The term scar tissue is often used to describe the process of new fibers binding together and joining the severed parts. Just as a scab is formed on the outer surface of the skin, so scar tissue is created below the skin encompassing all the layers of tissue cut through. We know that lymphatic vessels that were bisected in surgery will not heal up neatly and allow passage of lymphatic fluid to simply resume. These areas of scar tissue formation create physical obstructions that require the fluid to back-up and reroute. A more invasive surgery may result in larger chunks of lymphatic tissue being removed and could present a more serious challenge to recovery. Sometimes surgery also involves the removal of multiple lymph nodes and may sever larger collecting lymphatic vessels. Clearly, the more lymphatic tissue removed, the greater the risk for complications after surgery.

The process of removal of lymphatic fluid from the cellular environment involves a delicate balance of pressure gradients within the vessels, which allows fluid to move from an area of higher to one of lower osmotic pressure. It will begin to make sense that altered pressures within the vessels will change the direction of flow of the lymphatic fluid. The system by design moves fluid and metabolic products away from the cells towards the venous circulatory system, and towards the systems designed to remove waste matter from the body.

Though scar tissue is laid down fairly randomly, creating a roadblock to the movement of lymphatic fluid, we know that cryotherapy utilized after trauma promotes wound healing and prevents formation of excessive scar tissue (Block, Open Access J Sports Med). We also have evidence that manual lymph drainage in the area around wounds, promotes wound healing (Weiss, Phys Therapy). A reputable knowledge base already suggests that minimizing the inflammatory process as evidenced by tissue swelling, scar tissue formation, stagnation of fluid, and build up of trapped body heat in a surgical area, minimizes the stress on the involved tissue and promotes healing. The faster the flow of lymphatic fluid can resume by alternate pathways, the sooner the removal of waste products from the cellular environment can begin to occur, the better the recovery will proceed and the smaller the risk for complications will be.

Distinguishing Local and Non-local Swelling

Characteristically, the backflow of lymphatic fluid occurs distal to the site of the insult. The pathways have been interrupted and the fluid which cannot proceed on its usual forward route backs-up through the vessels into the surrounding tissue. We will use the term *local* swelling to differentiate the swelling which occurs at the site of injury, from *non-local* swelling which results from a backup of lymphatic fluid through the intact lymph vessels into the cellular environment where this fluid under normal circumstances originated.

Local swelling which can be temporary or become a low grade chronic condition, will generally be found right around the layers of tissue incised. This swelling will extend from a few millimeters to inches below the skin depending on the depth the surgical knife is required to penetrate. Unlike local swelling non-local swelling, which has its origin only a few millimeters below the skin where the superficial lymphatic system is disrupted, can back-up the length of an entire limb before spilling out into the interstitial space where it was first collected. The resulting distention of the skin can be painful, is cosmetically unflattering, often requires daily management, and without intervention the extent to which the tissue expands is limited only by the skin's elastic ability.

There is another simple identifying difference between local and non-local swelling that should inform the treating therapist and give pause to our consideration of how we choose to reduce swelling and support tissue healing. Typically, at the site of an injury or surgical incision, we find blood and lymphatic fluid mixing together as both vessel types are ruptured.

This may result in a dark brown or reddish bruising visible through the skin after injury, as blood and lymphatic fluid spill out of the vessels that usually carry them into the spaces between the cells. The discoloration of the skin is a result of tissue staining from the hemoglobin in the blood and can take days or even weeks to resolve. Contrastingly, the swelling found distal to the original site of trauma, the fluid that backs up into the tissue and causes tissue distention, will consist only of lymphatic fluid. This fluid is best described as viscous, it is light in appearance and can be whitish or yellowish on color. This fluid will not stain the skin.

There is yet another important distinguishing factor between local and non-local swelling. This distinction lies in the reason why fibrosis occurs. The formation of fibrosis is reparative after a surgical incision or trauma as incisions are naturally closed by the laying down of a collagen matrix. In non-local swelling fibrosis might be better described as a reactive process, where excess lymph fluid stagnates in the interstitium, thickening the tissue over time.

The reason for distinguishing between local and non-local swelling is to shed light on an important challenge facing the lymphedema community. We appear to bias the definition and management of lymphedema to non-local swelling, and there is no standard language or urgency of care for the management of local swelling. In trauma care, topical cooling and compression are commonly applied as first aid measures at the site of the injury to reduce local swelling, decrease the inflammatory response, decrease pain, and aid in tissue healing. Principles of wound healing inform us that the faster the inflammatory process is decreased, the less collagen will randomly be laid down, the less scar tissue will result.

Preventing Effect from Becoming Cause

Swelling is a natural occurrence after injury, one of the hallmarks of the inflammatory process, and an integral aspect of healing. One of the reasons for this natural mechanism is that if the swelling was the result of an accident, or if it was the result of a needed surgery, it forces us to stop moving to allow the body time to heal.

Yet why do orthopedic surgeons utilize cryotherapy in the operating room to begin reducing the swelling and inflammation right after surgery? We further have empirical evidence that cooling and compression not only reduce inflammation, swelling, and pain, but are associated with improved functional outcomes. Patients feel better and they heal faster.

In cancer-related surgical procedures involving the breast, such as in total or partial mastectomies and lumpectomies, managing the postoperative inflammatory process at the surgical site by cooling the tissue, something that is not commonly done, may well be the missed opportunity to promote more effective wound healing and prevent tissue changes, including scar tissue formation, that could have a progressive, destructive impact on the lymphatic system.

CHAPTER 4

A New Definition for Lymphedema

Inflammation – A New Perspective

If you have been a captive reader to this point, it will come as no surprise that I am about to recommend a new definition for lymphedema. The new definition puts the emphasis on the aspect of this condition we can impact right from the start. Inflammation is the hallmark of many diseases and the topic of discussion in health circles these days. What we now know is that inflammation in human tissue that is unchecked progresses overtime and sets up a condition we consider to be toxic to optimal health. An inflammatory process that is not stopped will expand its reach and ultimately disrupt a large system (Rakoff-Nahoum, The Yale Journal of Biology and Medicine). In medicine we already recognize that inflammatory processes can be low-grade and linger underground for a long time, sometimes for years, until they become visible to the eye and are then named by terms such as arthritis, coronary artery disease, neuropathies, a host of immune system diseases, cancer, and I believe, lymphedema too. Many of these emerging concepts about health are found in the realms of alternative and natural medicine and as yet remain contradicted from a strict scientific perspective. What is accepted is that during the time the low level inflammation is evolving, tissue damage occurs that has lasting impact on the functioning of the cells in the involved area. The movement in modern medicine is towards earlier detection of all inflammatory processes, before the irreversible damage is done. We are surprised when it takes years for the lymphedema to become evident. If we take the point of view that lymphedema can be defined as a low-grade inflammatory process before becoming evident, it will no longer come as a surprise that lymphedema suddenly appears. There is a reason why our mammoth immune system buckles and a disease becomes expressed. Like a giant army, the immune system does not just fall. More likely it falls after a good battle, in which cell by cell, it was taken over by an inflammatory process, an enemy that over time became formidable.

Inflammation in Lymphedema – A New Idea?

There is an obvious relationship between lymphedema and the immune system. Lymphatic dysfunction results in a disruption of the system that partakes in mitigating the vital immune response in the human body. The relationship between inflammation and the risk of infection is well understood: Inflammation predisposes to infection. It's not a far stretch to conclude that a condition of low grade inflammation in lymphatic tissue under the right circumstances can become a full blown infection. And that is exactly what we see when we witness yet another cellulitis infection so common in chronic lymphedema (Hutchinson, NLNLymphlink).

Interstitial edema as present in chronic lymphedema is simply edema expressing in between cells. Whenever it appears, edema is always an indication of an inflammatory response. Even in a low risk situation where there is no evidence yet of an infection, it should be understood as a vital immune system response. Prudence in medical care informs us to treat medically relevant signs at the first appearance. Current standards in lymphedema management geared to reducing the impact and consequences of chronic swelling are lymphatic drainage massage, compression bandaging and garments, and sequential pumping systems. Exercise, diet and skin care are also valuable tools in managing lymphedema. Though these are all essential and proven components of managing non-local lymphedema, none of the current standards assess or address the damage being done and currently left unchecked by unresolved local swelling.

Definition of Lymphedema

Old Definition:

Lymphedema is an accumulation of protein rich fluid in the interstitial space caused by physical damage to the lymphatic system resulting in a mechanical insufficiency or overload of the system, and a backup of lymphatic fluid into the interstitium. The stagnant fluid can have significant pathological and clinical consequences if left untreated. The swelling can affect any body part including the extremities, the face, the trunk, the abdomen or genital area.

New Definition:

Lymphedema is an accumulation of protein-rich fluid in the subcutaneous tissues caused by an inflammatory response that originates in physical damage to the lymphatic system *combined* with a resulting mechanical insufficiency or overload of the system. Lymphatic fluid backs up through the vessels and the accumulation of fluid in the interstitial space can have significant pathological and clinical consequences if left untreated. As with all potentially progressive inflammatory conditions, if treated at the onset, the risk of the condition becoming chronic, the damage to the system, the impact on functional status and quality of life, will be minimized.

A New Day in the Treatment of Lymphedema

Innovators run the risk of being ridiculed or admired. In the medical field new concepts require backing by scientific, double-blind, peer-reviewed research. Having completed an initial study on this topic still leaves many questions unanswered. Nevertheless, this place where more questions than answers exist, is a valuable well-source of creativity.

It will be no surprise to anyone knowledgeable of the division of labor in the medical field, that progress is sometimes hindered because the path of the clinician on the forefront of providing care, and that of the scientific researchers more often than not working behind the clinical screens, often do not cross. And so the intimate sharing of details that would facilitate the quickening of discovery is often not reached nearly fast enough to satisfy any of the parties, and certainly not our patients. Another humorous obstacle that keeps an imaginary divide between clinician and scientist, is that the two professions speak different languages. The clinician who is learning experientially in the clinic is often prone to subjective descriptions, while scientists prefer to remain in the realm of quantifiable measurements. Another frustrating aspect of scientific analysis to the practicing clinician is that two separate scientists exposed to the same facts may make contrasting interpretations, appearing to delay reaching a common conclusion the clinician would prefer to base a new treatment modality on.

To demonstrate the point in case, in the past years, two distinct scientific studies have demonstrated a correlation between inflammation and macrophages, one reporting that macrophages play an antifibrotic role in lymphedema (Ghanta, et al. American Journal of Physiology). Yet the second group of scientists cannot agree that long standing edema is sufficient to induce fibrosis and inflammation characteristic of human lymphedema (Markhus, et al. Arterioscler Thromb Vasc Biol). This conversation in the scientific community, circling around the exact meaning of the increased presence of macrophages in tissue with lymphedema and fibrosis, may well in the near future reveal evidence the scientific community requires in the direction of lymphedema being more urgently defined as an inflammatory response.

No matter the rate of progress, progress is being made. Clinical evidence already exists supporting that inflammation plays a role in the development of secondary lymphedema and that topical skin cooling has a therapeutic role in resolving the symptoms of inflammation. This evidence also supports the unfolding rationale that lymphedema may well be more accurately defined as an inflammatory process combined with a mechanical insufficiency, and that patients with lymphedema would be better served by more aggressive anti-inflammatory management.

CHAPTER 5

Topical Skin Cooling as The First Step in Treatment

What Cooling Does

Cooling for lymphedema you will come to see, is a valuable addition to any program geared to managing this swelling. The purpose of skin cooling over lymphedematous areas is to reduce the skin temperature, which reduces tissue pressure and inflammation in the superficial layers of the skin where the superficial lymphatics reside, and where the back-up of secondary lymphedema occurs. The known theoretical effect is created by a rapid collapse of the arterioles impacted by the cooling medium and results in fluid exiting the targeted area. A benefit of cooling and the resulting rapid decrease in tissue pressure to the lymphedema specialist is that underlying scar tissue and fibrotic patches become more readily palpable, allowing fibrosis management techniques to begin immediately and be more targeted.

The term fibrosis is used to describe the formation of excess fibrous connective tissue in a reparative or reactive process. In non-local lymphedema the formation of fibrosis is best described as a reactive process, and identifies hardened areas under the skin where the protein rich lymph fluid becomes thickened over time. The progression and staging of lymphedema is measured by the level of fibrosis and rigidity present in the tissue. Fibrotic areas, once formed, will not resolve without treatment. Fibrosis further complicates the movement of lymphatic fluid, and is cause to progression of the disease of lymphedema.

The use of cryotherapy in the reduction of inflammation in human tissue, either post operatively or in traumatic injury, also has its opponents. Surface cooling of human tissue at or below subzero temperatures for an extended period is a known cause of tissue ischemia and long lasting damage to the microvasculature. Those who oppose also argue against reducing the natural inflammatory response and interfering with a physiological process which under normal circumstances is uniquely geared to healing tissue injury. Scientific inquiry revealing the pathway by which excessive vasoconstriction reduces the flow of oxygen to cells is allowing us to gain new insight. Studies have already revealed the pathway by which the myogenic muscle tone in humans is impacted as the Rho-kinase pathway. A recent study (Christmas et al, Microvasc. Res.) revealed that cryotherapy influences this pathway and contributes to vascular vasoconstriction during and following cryotherapy treatment in humans. It is known (Yao et al, J Cardiovasc. Res.) that abnormal activation of the Rho-kinase pathway in the cardiovascular system unbalances the production of vasodilating and vasoconstricting substances. Though it is known that this pathway is involved in regulating myogenic tone and lymphatic pump activity in non-human studies (Hosaka, Mizuno, Ohhashi, American Physiological Society), what is not yet known is how the Rho-kinase pathway is involved in lymphatic pump activity in humans. We also do not yet know how to modify this pathway for possible therapeutic repair of lymphatic pump failure.

The Evidence

Over the years my patients encouraged me to share the results of my successful cooling experiments. The idea began to grow that I might produce a scientific study to satisfy the medical community that topical skin cooling had merit as a treatment modality in the clinical management of lymphedema. I was fortunate to make contact with Dr. Harvey Mayrovitz who already had extensive knowledge of lymphedema and had published many scientific studies on the topic. At our first meeting I gave anecdotal evidence of the cooling technique I had incorporated into the lymphedema therapy session. Dr. Mayrovitz was surprised and curious. I will forever be grateful that he agreed to lend his expertise.

The result is a study titled *Local Skin Cooling as an Aid to the Management of Patients with Breast Cancer-Related Lymphedema and Fibrosis of the Arm or Breast* (Mayrovitz, Yzer, Lymphology 50(2017)56-66). We were able to show that topical surface cooling of lymphedematous and fibrotic regions leads to a softening of tissue as measured by local indentation forces. In the discussion portion of our completed study we explained the reasoning behind the hardness reduction that occurs when cooling lymphedematous tissue, and we presented an analysis of the clinical significance of this important finding. We were not yet able to isolate the specific cooling related mechanism with 100% certainty as this was difficult due to the range of effects associated with tissue cooling that include hemodynamic, neuromuscular and metabolic.

It is worth commenting here that much remains unknown about the lymphatic system. More is known about the blood vascular system than the lymphatic system. We do not know yet what the actual impact of moderate topical cooling is on the lining of the lymphatic vessel. How does moderate cooling impact the lymphatic endothelial cell? How does moderate cooling as defined in this book influence the lymphatic pump?

How Cooling Works

The main hemodynamic effect of topical skin cooling is believed to be a reduction in blood flow associated with cold induced arteriolar vasoconstriction (Khoshnevis, et al. J Biomech Eng). Vessel constriction reduces fluid transport into the interstitium and also decreases venous intravascular pressure and likely explains the reduction in indentation resistance we noted with the instruments used for measuring tissue pressure. In the study I co-authored and reference, we were not able to confirm that skin water percentage was actually reduced. The likely reason for this is that only one set of measurements was collected from each subject during a treatment session. However, over the course of treatment, all subjects showed decreases in girth measurement, a standard method used in the clinical management of lymphedema for defining progress. Another benefit of cooling over lymphedematous swelling is the resulting decrease in superficial skin temperature. In an area of fluid congestion this adds the benefit of decreasing the likeliness of bacterial growth, a known risk in chronic lymphedema.

Even though scientific inquiry has not yet confirmed the exact mechanisms by which cooling impacts lymphedema, what is clear, is that cooling therapy within the moderate temperature range adopted in the study, penetrating and altering the temperature and movement of fluid in the superficial layers of the skin, results in the therapeutic effect of decreasing tissue pressure, allowing the therapist to more rapidly improve the presenting symptoms of pain, swelling and decreased mobility. And that is what people living with lymphedema need, treatment options that efficiently and reliably reduce tissue fluid and decrease the risk of lymphedema progressing.

Clinical Significance

This is where I share the practical benefits of this treatment modality to people living with lymphedema. When cooling is applied to a targeted area, there is cooling related softening of tissue that results, while pressure on sensory nerve endings is partially or fully relieved. For patients who have fibrosis related nerve compression pain, this manifests as a reduction in pain that is rapidly achieved without the use of medications. For a physical therapist there is no better reward than to hear your patient say "My pain is gone." When tissue pressure is decreased, muscles and muscle spindles in those areas where lymphedema and fibrosis were impacting muscle function is improved. When the communication between the peripheral nerves and the central nervous system normalizes, there is an increased ability of the muscles to contract, improving range of movement, muscle strength, and thus function. Can you see me jumping for joy? These are the goals of rehabilitation. Less swelling, less pain, more movement, more function, and better quality of life!

Though topical skin cooling is not intended to replace the need for lymphatic drainage massage, it has been my observation that it reduces the amount of time needed to manually clear a targeted area. Though this may vary by patient and by therapist, a 50% reduction in time was common. Clinically this allows the clinician to more effectively utilize therapy time for fibrosis management and therapeutic activities. Topical skin cooling can also easily be carried over in the home giving patients more independence in managing symptoms. Lymphedema clinicians may not realize how elitist our clinical standards for lymphedema management are until they have the opportunity to venture into third world countries where trained specialists and lymphedema supplies do not exist. It is for this reason too, that topical skin cooling for lymphedema holds potential as a cost-effective and accessible treatment option in the management of patients with lymphedema worldwide.

How to Cool

Topical skin cooling can easily and safely be done in the clinic or home. Immerse a washcloth or small towel in a bowl of ice water, wring it out, and contour the affected body part. Once the cloth towels warm up, which may happen quickly since skin temperatures over lymphedematous areas may be slightly higher due to a buildup of body heat, immerse the towels in the cool water, wring them out, and reapply. This process is repeated until the skin cools, the towels no longer warm up, and the tissue pressure decreases slightly to palpation. The rule of thumb in applying cold to sensitive areas of the body is to stay within comfort level. If the first contact with the cold washcloth is jarring, add room temperature water to the ice water mixture to reduce the temperature and impact. The treatment is effective in reducing body heat as long as the temperature of the ice water mixture is colder than the skin temperature. The resulting change may be slight or more evident depending on the level of fluid and heat buildup present in the tissue.

When applying topical skin cooling for treating lymphedema the therapeutic goal is achieved by cooling the skin an average of 13.8°C or 25°F. This correlates to a change in human skin temperature from an average baseline of 32.7°C or 91°F to a low of 18.9°C or 66°F. Since the cooling applied is moderate, the actual change in temperature is brief, and the skin temperature immediately begins to rise again. The lymphatic system is easily impacted by a slight change in temperature, be it an increase or decrease in temperature, as the lymphatic vessels are located close to the surface of the skin. There is no therapeutic value to increasing the temperature over lymphedematous skin as increased temperatures correlate to increased metabolism and increased swelling. There is however now proven therapeutic value to decreasing the skin temperature as suggested here, for managing the symptoms of lymphedema.

The drawback of the treatment as described is that ice water placed in a bowl can spill, increasing the risk of slippage and falls. And cooling the involved body part while lying on a bed causes the bedding to get wet. For home cooling and even for use in the clinic, I have created a less messy option using cooling towels which are the PVA chamois sports towels popularized in recent years. You can find a resource for these towels online, on my website or pick them up locally. The cooling towels need to be wet, wrung out, and placed in the refrigerator in a moisture retaining bag. Cooling towels are not to be placed in the freezer as they will dry out and become hardened, have no therapeutic value and could damage your skin upon contact. Frozen objects such as ice or commercially available gel packs, should never be placed directly on the skin to avoid injury. A damp cooling towel, once chilled in the refrigerator, is the right temperature to place on the lymphedematous body part and achieve changes in baseline skin temperature as listed above. Cooling towels retain cold almost as well as cloth washcloths as they are made of absorbent PVA, Polyvinyl Alcohol, material. Have several cooling cloths chilled in the refrigerator to apply in sequence. It is also possible to cool cloth washcloths or towels in the refrigerator. Wet and wring them out and place in a moisture retaining bag until use. If the cooling towels warm up quickly after placement on the body this is an indication of how much heat was trapped in the superficial skin layers. Trapped body heat is one of the symptoms of unmanaged lymphedema. It causes a rise in temperature within the lymphatic fluid, the lining of the lymphatic vessels and within the cellular environment. It is one of the markers of low-grade inflammation and one of the conditions for a buildup of a festering chronic inflammation in tissue. Removing this trapped body heat by applying topical cooling prevents the inflammatory process from advancing and the disease process from progressing.

Cooling towels can be applied as often as needed to help manage the symptoms of lymphedema. During the summer months and in warmer climates, when body temperature and cellular metabolism are increased, this treatment is particularly beneficial. With regular use the involved body part will become softer and your skin more supple. These are indications of lymphedema being better controlled! Topical skin cooling is best used in conjunction with other components of a lymphedema program as directed by the lymphedema therapist. The suggested sequence is to cool the involved tissue first, perform self-manual lymphatic massage or apply a pneumatic pumping treatment, followed by the application of various bandaging and compression methods and exercises as prescribed.

Indications/ Contraindications/Precautions to Cooling

Contraindications and precautions to the use of moderate topical skin cooling are few. Precautions include an intolerance to moderate cold temperatures caused by an incompetent nervous system, or the complete absence of temperature sensation. There is no risk of physical damage to human tissue or the important microvasculature when the skin is cooled to an average of 13.8°C or 25°F below normal skin temperatures. Open wounds are a clear contraindication, as infection could result and the sensitive germinating wound bed could be disrupted, further delaying wound healing.

Unlike manual lymphatic drainage, topical skin cooling as defined, is not contraindicated in an acute cellulitis infection. *Immediate referral to an MD for emergency medical management is of the essence, and this recommendation should not be taken lightly.*

Cooling over an infected area removes the trapped body heat that typically allows the invading organisms to rapidly multiply. Topical skin cooling supports the goals of emergency management of trauma and infection where cooling packs are applied to stem swelling, reduce infection, and reduce pain. *Topical skin cooling by drawing heat out of tissue also prevents the buildup of heat that commonly leads to cellulitis infections and may well be a valuable tool in deterring this common infection.*

Topical skin cooling which decreases human skin temperature an average of 13.8°C or 25°F does not ever approximate the freezing temperatures that commercially available cooling gel packs attain. The moderate cold temperature suggested for use in the topical cooling of lymphedematous skin does not cause any damage to the microvasculature of the superficial lymphatics. Besides staying in the safe temperature zone it is also advisable to apply cooling within the patient's tolerance. If the ice water feels too cold, adding room temperature water to lessen the initial contact will increase comfort and still provide therapeutic impact. In the clinic, surface temperature of ice water or cooling cloths can be measured with an infrared thermometer.

CHAPTER 6

Testimonials

Introduction to The Testimonials

Testimonials have a place in the evolution of any new treatment method. Though in the medical field where empirical evidence rules, they are generally received with no more than a grain of salt, they at least begin to open our minds to the possibility of something we previously did not know. Testimonials when delivered live give the recipient the benefit of using auditory and visual senses to not only hear the message but to observe body language allowing the collection of data to fuel the initial acceptance or rejection of the testimony. A written testimony has the disadvantage of being one dimensional and not revealing of auditory or visual clues. I can tell you that the three patients mentioned below are real, and they are amongst the many patients I have treated with topical skin cooling over the past 10 years.

Dionne – Lymphedema of The Arm and Breast

Dionne's story touched me deeply from the start. She was diagnosed with breast cancer as a young bride. She was very much in love with her husband and decided from the onset that she would not have her breasts removed even though the recommendation was for a double mastectomy and reconstruction, and even though her cancer was advanced when it was first discovered. As Dionne described it to me, "My breasts are not only a part of me, but they are a part of my marriage to my husband. If I don't absolutely have to lose them, I don't want to lose them." The surgeon reluctantly agreed to perform a lumpectomy before more invasive surgery but Dionne had to agree to more aggressive treatment which included a larger than usual dosage of radiation therapy. She had radiation therapy daily for four months and as a result Dionne developed swelling in her involved breast. Because she was motivated to succeed, she got herself into lymphedema therapy and on an exercise program as soon as she physically could. She found her way to my clinic where I noted the increased temperature of the involved breast. We began cooling her swollen breast with cold washcloths to draw the buildup of heat out of her tissue. The improvement was fast. She observed with a sigh of relief at the end of the first session that her involved breast was softer and the feelings of heat, pressure and pain under the skin were lessened. I did not have to convince her to keep cooling the affected area at home. Today, seven years after the initial diagnosis and her lumpectomy, she is on a cooling program, she exercises regularly and watches her diet closely. She remains healthy and is still happily in love.

Her decision to go against the surgeon's recommendation to have a double mastectomy may not be the right decision for everyone. Her story does clearly show however, the value of questioning any medical opinion and making the one that is best for you.

Sally – Lymphedema of the Trunk

Sally's story will sound familiar to many who saw their lymphedema show up years after the original surgery occurred. Patients whose lymphatic system have been disrupted are always told that they are at risk for lymphedema and that it can come on even years down the road. In those cases it may especially seem that the lymphedema arose out of the blue. Sometimes we can point to a life changing circumstance that shifted the balance in the body. Let's hear Sally's story.

Sally had a total mastectomy without reconstruction 17 years prior to us meeting each other. She reported that she had no symptoms of lymphedema during those years. I want to state here, that I cannot be sure the swelling wasn't slowly developing and would have been evident earlier to an experienced eye. But there is no doubt that two years prior to walking into my clinic Sally's life changed. Her adult son died suddenly in a fatal motor vehicle accident. Sally described the stress and emotional pain this caused her and the impact it had on her health. One of the consequences she reported, was that she developed lymphedema in her chest and arm. This mother's pain was unimaginable. Her swelling also settled into the rib cage below the site of the mastectomy. Her knowledgeable doctor referred her to a lymphedema clinic where she received lymphatic drainage massage and compression wrapping. She reported to me that the swelling in her arm and chest wall were made manageable with the caring therapy she received, but she continued to complain to her doctor about a discomfort in the rib cage below the surgical site. A rib fracture or metastases were ruled out. Lymphedema therapists are often respectfully amused that the worse possible diagnosis is often considered before the simplest.

Of course for purposes of my testimonials, I have to pick cases that responded exceptional to topical skin cooling to make a teaching point. This is never done with intention to discredit any of my colleagues, but to add knowledge. When I evaluated Sally I could see that the rib cage on the involved side where she had her symptoms was more distended than the uninvolved. To the untrained eye that may appear to be additional fatty tissue lodged in the area, but from experience I knew there was likely some fluid pocketed in between the ribs, putting pressure on sensory nerve endings signaling pain to the brain. Sometimes secondary lymphedema originating in the breast drains into the superficial lymphatics located below the breast, over the ribcage and may even at times present as abdominal swelling and distention, leaving the patient thinking that they are just gaining weight. I can't tell you how often I have heard untreated swelling referred to as increased weight by the unaware patient. On that first visit, I performed cooling therapy over the targeted area in addition to applying fibrosis techniques in between the involved ribs. We completed the treatment with manual lymph drainage and myofascial stretching, and by the end of the first session Sally said that the pain and pressure had almost disappeared. I cautioned Sally that the swelling might return since it had been there for a period of time. We created a personalized home program just for her. I still speak to Sally from time to time to check up on her. The swelling never returned as it had before I treated her and she credits cooling and exercise for that. But from time to time she reports an increase in pressure, indicative of mild swelling, in the area. As a result of her time spent in therapy Sally also decided to enhance her exercise program and she took up swimming. The arm movements associated with swimming strokes proved to be particularly helpful for her to strengthen her upper body and keep her ribs clear from pooling of fluid. Sally is very happy that she has her life back!

Maria – Lymphedema of the Leg

Maria's story is different than the previous two. She developed ovarian cancer at the age of 61 and reported that her lymphedema started 3 years after her surgeries and treatments were completed. When she arrived at my clinic she had been living with lymphedema for 5 years and was knowledgeable of all the traditional treatment options. She was already quite the model patient. She utilized a compression pump, she wore compression garments during the day or sometimes applied multi-layer bandaging, she used a custom night time compression garment, and she made sure to visit her lymphedema therapist twice a year for a course of treatment to keep the swelling under control. She was doing everything we could ask of our patients.

As with many people who live with lymphedema, Maria described a process of increased buildup of pressure and heat in the affected limb during the day, especially during the summer months, even while wearing a Class II compression stocking. And she noticed a softening of her limb at night after applying her compression pump, and sleeping in a nighttime compression garment. People with chronic lymphedema often describe a buildup of warmth or heat in the limb during the activity of the day when movement and metabolism are at a peak. Especially on a warm summer day, this buildup can lead to a sensation of burning inside in the limb. Cooling is particularly helpful in such cases as a cold washcloth or cooling towel will immediately begin to draw the heat out of the superficial lymphatic system and decrease the skin temperature. At the first treatment Maria noticed that cooling made an impact on the discomfort she regularly experienced from the buildup of pressure and heat in her limb. She has now added cooling of the limb to her lymphedema treatment, fitting it in with all other aspects of her program.

Closing Statements to Testimonials

If the above testimonials created more questions than answers, then we are on the right track. This is exactly how I felt when I first started using topical skin cooling. My own distrust that this simple treatment could be so effective prevented me initially from seeking scientific rationale to explain what I was observing. Sharing the testimonials and research available to date, and enlisting you as co-investigators is the next step in spreading the word and building confidence in a treatment method that by its ease of use and its effectiveness, belongs in the rank of first-stop treatments for lymphedema.

CHAPTER 7

For Lymphedema Therapists

If you specialize in treating lymphedema, this chapter is for you! Helping a patient take control of an illness and disability is a humbling experience. And often it's the small things we do, a smile, words of encouragement, or even a simple treatment idea, that go a long way in supporting the journey from illness back to health. One possible reason that topical skin cooling has not yet been considered for use in treating lymphedema is that this swelling shows up in temperature sensitive areas of the human body where applying traditional cryotherapy could lead to discomfort, burns, pain and microvasculature damage.

I guarantee you that I am not about to teach you anything radically new. Topical skin cooling is not a novel treatment to you. After reading this you may even wonder why you had not thought of its utility in the management of lymphedema. At the National Lymphedema conference in 2016, where I co-presented a poster on the completed study, I discussed this treatment modality with a lymphedema therapist who admitted to me in confidence that she regularly placed cooling gel packs on top of the multi-layer bandaging at the end of her lymphedema treatment session. She said that it had just made sense to her that diffused cooling would have therapeutic impact on the superficial lymphatic system, and her patients loved the cooling effect that filtered through the cloth bandages onto their limbs. We had a good chuckle and decided we would call ourselves "the Coolers", as if part of a secret pact.

Experienced therapists have good instincts about their patients need. New treatment ideas are developed from this intuitive knowing. Yet therapists tend to be such a humble group. Until recently we have been a group comprised mostly of women, who notoriously do not toot their own horns. We are more prone to follow than invent new treatment methods based on our intuitive insights. In writing this book I take a stand not only for my patients but for female therapists. Since our desire is to be of service we can help our patients one at a time, as they come to us, or we can help a whole population by bringing forth creative treatment ideas. If I found one female therapist who already intuitively uses cooling gel packs in treating lymphedema, then how many more are out there? And how many more new treatment ideas are waiting to be revealed?

How to Cool in the Clinic

The Lymphedema Therapy Clinic is the ideal center for patient evaluation, treatment and education. A model clinic should offer access to all commonly used treatment modalities available for lymphedema and assist the patient in creating the optimal individualized program. A modality proven effective for one may not be the best choice for another.

When applying topical skin cooling for lymphedema the concerns that need to be addressed are **skin contact, effectiveness, and safe temperature range.**

Skin Contact and Effectiveness

The superficial lymphatic system is located in the surface layers of the skin. When applying topical skin cooling the goal is to cover the skin in the targeted area with cold cloths or cooling towels to remove body heat trapped in the lymphatic fluid and in the surrounding tissue. As a result the tissue pressure decreases and the skin softens. In our study, we took skin temperature readings with an infrared skin thermometer before and after cooling, and tissue pressure readings with a tissue pressure reader, before and after applying topical skin cooling. You do not need to have these instruments present to perform the treatment. With a little practice you can palpate changes in skin temperature and tissue pressure before and after cooling. Having an infrared skin thermometer to experiment with would offer objective feedback about the change in temperature before and after treatment.

Select a towel that contours best to the shape and size of the targeted body part. That body part could be a breast, arm or armpit, a thigh etc. I started using washcloths in the clinic as they were easily dipped in ice water and light enough to wring out by hand, and contour to curved areas. For a larger body part a hand size towel may be more user friendly. For my comfort I preferred to use household dishwashing gloves for immersing my hands in cold water.

Another product that is readily available and contours well to the body surface is a cooling towel. Cooling towels have been popularized for use in sports. They are lightweight and designed to hold moisture and create a cooling effect. There is a special angle of use I developed for use in topical skin cooling. Wet the cooling towel, wring it out and place it in a moisture retaining bag in the refrigerator. By cooling this PVA fabric in the refrigerator, *not* the freezer, the cooling towel is effective in decreasing human skin temperature the recommended 13.8°C or 25°F needed to impact the superficial lymphatic and reduce superficial swelling. Once removed from refrigeration the PVA cooling towel does not maintain the attained cold temperature very long but it effectively wicks away body heat trapped in the superficial layers. I recommend preparing several cooling towels in advance and using them in sequence to create the same effect as the washcloths dipped in cold water. This method is desirable for home use.

Safe temperature range

The temperature required to achieve the desired therapeutic effect in the superficial layers of the skin where the delicate lymphatics reside is described as *moderate* and decreases human skin temperature an average of 13.8°C or 25°F. This moderate temperature change is at least 30 degrees above freezing and does not put the patient or the delicate microvasculature structure at any risk. Average human skin temperature is 32.7°C or 91°F and a cold washcloth dipped in ice water or a cooling towel out of the refrigerator applied to the skin, will result in an approximately 13.8°C or 25°F skin temperature change after several applications, decreasing skin temperature to a low of 18.9°C or 66°F. *Never* use ice or commercially available gel-packs directly on the skin when using the cooling application for lymphedema as freezing temperatures, even when applied through a protective cloth cover, could damage the microvasculature. Conventional gel packs and cryocuff machines used in therapy clinics are designed to cool to depths up to 3 cm below the skin, a depth unnecessary for managing lymphedema that puts the microvasculature at risk of permanent damage due to being subjected to extreme and even freezing temperatures.

Clinical Relevance

Clinical therapists are always concerned with managing treatment time and achieving functional therapy goals while applying optimal standards of care. You will be pleased to know that topical skin cooling positively impacts your treatment by allowing you to achieve a reduction of swelling in a shorter amount of available therapy time. Once you observe how tissue swelling and firmness respond to the application of cooling within the safe temperature guidelines provided, you will be as surprised and pleased as I was. Sometimes less is better. In the case of impacting the delicate superficial lymphatic system, less cold is indeed more effective and has therapeutic impact while extreme cold damages lymphatic tissue. In the clinical study the cooling was followed by a short sequence of lymphatic drainage massage and the application of compression bandaging. In addition tissue lengthening techniques, muscle strengthening exercises and fibrosis management were started on the first day of treatment. The patient was also instructed in self bandaging on the first day of care, beginning the process of instilling confidence and self-reliance in their ability to manage their own symptoms. If your patient is in pain, you will be particularly pleased that the pain level will almost immediately recede after applying topical skin cooling as the pressure on nerve endings embedded in the tissue, is quickly reduced. When the swelling has been present for a while, we can be sure that overtime, the linings of the lymphatic vessels have become irritated and inflamed. Reducing the inflammation and removing trapped heat in these vessels will allow the cell wall linings to begin to heal again. Theoretically, this correlates to improving the function of the lymph vessels.

Previously you might have started your treatment session with a lymphatic drainage massage. It has been my observation that the lymphedema therapy session often becomes overpowered by the lymphatic drainage massage and the application of compression bandaging. This allows proportionally little to no time for rehabilitation goals that include muscle strengthening and achieving functional goals. Once you begin the treatment session by applying topical skin cooling you will require less time for lymphatic massage and will advance more easily to fibrosis techniques and functional range of motion and therapy goals. Be sure to instruct your patients on day one in the technique of compression wrapping. It is not as impossible as many therapists think. By allowing the beautiful human being in front of you to become independent in managing their own symptoms they can more readily have a full healing and return to claiming purposeful lives.

As lymphedema therapists, we need to take a step back and remind ourselves what is important to our patients. If there is a more effective way to achieve a goal, in this case reducing and preventing swelling caused by secondary lymphedema, why would we not include it? And if we can make our patient more independent in managing their own symptoms, why would we not? These are exactly the benefits topical skin cooling offers to the management of lymphedema. A more effective way to give our patients the outcomes and independence they want.

Add to the Knowledge Base

Topical skin cooling is commonly used to treat swelling post trauma but has not yet found a place in the management of lymphedema. I believe this is because lymphedema therapists do not see patients with acute swelling, nor are we routinely summoned to the recovery bed of a patient after breast surgery to begin preventative care. We are also not present when the bandages are first removed from the surgical site in the surgeon's office. We rarely get to intervene in the management of what I have coined local swelling: Swelling that results from the initial trauma and inflammation caused by the cancer related surgical procedure. Based on my experience I am convinced that in these early stages postoperatively lie a greater opportunity to reduce lingering inflammation and positively impact the formation of scar tissue. These are both factors that influence how long the swelling lingers in the tissue potentially creating obstructions to the flow of lymphatic fluid. In cancer-related procedures where lymphedema is a risk factor, medical professionals have already made the case that preoperative education plays a role in preventing lymphedema (Simmons, Holly, Nursing and Health). And now we have more knowledge and evidence that early management of inflammation may play a role in preventing the onset of secondary lymphedema.

CHAPTER 8

Living on Purpose in Spite of Lymphedema

At a time when the crucial relationship between our mind and body to health has become better understood, and we have evidence of the intrinsic connection between emotional well-being and the immune system, this chapter on living on purpose is of great value. Though I cannot do the subject justice in one chapter, I can give an introduction that may begin to change the way you look at your health.

"Thoughts are things" has been a popular saying in metaphysics and philosophy and, now it would appear, even science is chiming in. While wisdom teachings of the ages have contemplated, studied, and taught these principles, more recently science has provided supportive evidence that the chemicals inside our bodies form a dynamic information network that link the mind and body.

Neuropeptides are signaling molecules involved in many physiological functions that originate in the central nervous system (Burbach, JP, Methods Mol Biol). These substrates have been proven to communicate with receptors on vital immune cells participating in the body's immune response (Pert, Candace, Molecules of Emotion). Scientists are helping us to understand that there is a biomechanical basis for our emotions, and that our emotions impact our personal world and influence how we experience and create our lives.

My patients have taught me valuable lessons. Tragedy breaks us out of apathy. Tragedy often comes unexpected and reminds us that our time here is not guaranteed. It spurs us into action that can help realize our dreams. Sometimes it takes loss of health, even loss of life of someone we love, to remind us what we hold dear and what we want to experience in this one precious life. Tragedy can serve to get us back on track, it can remind us that a life lived on purpose is actually the more exciting, dynamic, and fulfilling life.

What is Your Purpose in Life?

So, what is it that is calling you? What has your illness made you aware of that you would like to do, that you *must* do? Here is an exercise to help you organize your thoughts and ideas about your purpose.

To prepare for this exercise, open a notebook to a fresh page and draw a line down the center.

Make sure you will not be interrupted for 30 minutes. Get quiet, take a few centering breaths, close your eyes, and ask yourself, "If there were no obstacles to achieving my dreams, what is it that I would want to do?" Write down whatever comes to mind, do not edit! Do your best to remove any thoughts of limitation from the vision in your mind. In reality we all have limitations, the point is to learn to move around them. Limitations do not have to define us. For right now, dream as big as you can, and let your heart sing its song freely. Write down as many things as come to mind! Luxuriate in your dreams.

When the list is complete, answer the following question for each of the dreams you wrote. What is the first step, even if only a small step, that needs to happen for dream number 1 to begin to fulfill, for dream number 2 to begin to fulfill, etc? It may be something as simple as telling someone your dream, researching your dream, or buying a new book on a topic of interest. Make sure you write at least one action step down for every dream.

Even though you may not have the faintest idea how your dreams could actually come through, you will have voiced them and you will have indicated a beginning step on the path to achieving them. You have now opened the door in your mind to the possibility of your dream becoming real at some point in the future. Place this worksheet where you will see it often, even copy it and place several copies around your living space. My suggestion is that you look at it daily. Interact with it. Color or doodle on it, add notes as they arise and take any small action steps you can! Allow the pathway, that groove in your mind where the dream lives, to deepen just a little more every time you read the notes or take an action step. Believe that in some mysterious way you have begun the process of breathing life into one or more of your dreams.

Obstacles to Living Your Purpose After Cancer

If you have secondary lymphedema, the kind of lymphedema that results from surgeries, then you likely have a current or past diagnosis of cancer. No doubt a daunting diagnosis. Lymphedema should not be the obstacle to achieving your purpose in life. Neither should cancer. Though a diagnosis of cancer has the ability to put your plans on hold and maybe even change them, never ever give up on your goals. You will know that you are back in control of your life when you can, in one breath, say that you may have been touched by cancer, but that you still believe in your dreams. Never take no for an answer. There are always opportunities and possibilities to make a dream become reality.

Make a decision to tell yourself daily that no matter what is occurring, *you* are the commander of your life and *you* command your life with absolute authority. Repeat this sentence until you feel it as real. Allow the power of belief to build within you.

There is a place within all of us that puts us in a receptive mode for healing. I describe it as the greatest position of self-love we can get to. You will know it when you can feel hope, confidence, and self-love rising from the core of your being reminding you once again you are here to live, love, and create!

The Next Step

Getting your lymphedema managed will give you extra time to put towards your purposeful goals. A well-planned daily program will help keep lymphedema in check so that it will not interfere with your life.

Now is the time to review how you habitually live your life and care for yourself. Consider your eating habits, exercise, work and career, family relations, social life, and stress management. You may want to write the list down and score each area on a scale from 1 to 10, with 10 being the highest level of satisfaction. No one book can provide you with all the tools to re-create yourself. Begin with the areas that call to you the most, realizing that you can easily juggle several of them. No reason you can't begin an exercise program and change your eating habits at the same time, since that combination is also going to have a wonderful impact on your stress levels. I have found that once I set new intentions and begin to take action in the direction of the desired outcome that things show up. I find course offers in my email, I get an unexpected call from a friend, it is as if I am following an intuitive knowing to assist myself in achieving my desired goal.

The process is put into motion when you decide what your next step is. It is up to you to decide, and then begin taking steps, no matter how small the steps may seem to you. Will you trust me on this? Start walking in the direction of your dreams!

I would totally be remiss if I did not mention the great benefit of quiet time to health and to our ability to sort things out. Meditation or contemplation can easily be learned. Learning to still the mind from outer and inner distractions allows us to focus our attention. Utilizing quiet time to reduce distractions is a priceless skill. Contemplative practice is the first thing I turn to when I feel I am becoming overwhelmed by events and thoughts in my head. It allows me to reclaim control, and refocus my mind on my higher goals. It is how I wrote this book, one focused word at a time.

Please accept my invitation at the end of the book to join me in the Facebook group where I will continue to post helpful tips on living a purposeful life.

CHAPTER 9

Frequently Asked Questions

Risk Reductions Factors for Lymphedema

The National Lymphedema Network, NLN, has published a position paper on lymphedema risk-reduction practices which is available on its website at www.lymphnet.org. I invite you to visit and download the position paper. The main points are included below.

Skin care

Since the surface of the skin can be the entry point for intruding bacteria that may cause infection and exacerbate swelling, good skin care is important. Avoid cuts, sunburns, insect bites, and readily clean all scratches or punctures with soap and water. Observe for signs of infection such as redness, increased temperature, rash, or itching. Cellulitis, which is the general term used for an infection of the cells, is a serious medical condition requiring immediate care and treatment from a medical doctor. It is recommended to avoid puncture such as injections or blood draws, and even blood pressure readings on the involved limb.

Use of compression

Your lymphedema specialist will assist you in establishing a compression program that best suits your lifestyle and specific presentation of lymphedema. Use of compression during the day helps to keep the swelling at the lowest possible level. You may require an elastic garment for your arms or legs. Or you may require a compression bra, or specialized compression garment for the trunk, neck or head. Your therapist may refer you to a medical supplier for fitting. Multi-layer compression bandaging is an excellent tool to help keep your swelling controlled. Learning how to apply the bandages may initially seem like a daunting task, but will provide you with independence in managing the fluctuations in swelling common in living with lymphedema. You may benefit from a pneumatic compression device, also called a lymphedema pump.

Activities and lifestyle choices

As with any recovery process, it is suggested that you gradually build up the duration and intensity of activity. Monitor the involved extremity during and after a new exercise program for any changes. Since weight gain impacts lymphedema, maintaining optimal weight is an important aspect in managing lymphedema. Remember even with lymphedema the daily recommended water intake is half your bodyweight in ounces. Avoid *extremes* of temperature, both cold and heat, as either can damage microvasculature and further exacerbate lymphedema. The topical skin cooling as recommended utilizes moderate cold temperatures which are defined within the body of the book and never approach freezing. Never use ice or a frozen gel pack directly on your skin as it will cause ice burns.

Air Travel and Lymphedema

Even though the cabin is pressurized during air travel, if you have a compromised lymphatic system, there is increased risk for lymphedema to be triggered. Fluid that leaks out of lymphatic vessels into the cellular environment can result in rapid swelling and cause great distress. Individuals with a diagnosis of lymphedema, as well as individuals at high risk for developing lymphedema, are recommended to wear a compression garment on the affected body part during air travel. A compression garment supports the individual by applying an external, graded force to the affected area. Take frequent walks in the aisle of the airplane, obtain assistance for lifting heavy luggage, drink plenty of water, and wear a compression garment during the entire flight.

Exercise and Lymphedema

One of the most exciting developments I have seen as a lymphedema therapist over the past 10 years is the change in knowledge and attitude regarding the use and benefit of exercise and resistance training in managing secondary lymphedema (Rehana L. Ahmed et al. Journal of Clinical Oncology). We now have scientific evidence that strengthening muscles with resistance does not impact lymphedema negatively (McKenzie, Kalda, Journal of Clinical Oncology). The opposite is true, stronger muscles help to mobilize lymphatic fluid towards reentry into the venous circulatory system. As with all new physical exercise training programs, one must gradually build up the use of resistance. It is recommended that a compression garment be worn during exercise to support the area impacted by lymphedema.

If you exercise with lymphedema I can offer a few practical suggestions. You might want to keep an older compression garment handy to wearing during exercise so that the newer one is clean for use after you exercise. Make sure the compression value it still within a good range. My patients who exercise regularly have found that cooling the affected area right after helps to resolve any increase in swelling that may occur due to increased metabolism. The production of lymphatic fluid is known to increase with dynamic exercise and can result in a feeling of increased fullness. Wearing a well fitting compression garment and cooling right after exercise will aid in a faster recovery.

When you are ready to resume an exercise program, allow your rehabilitation and lymphedema specialist to guide you in making wise exercise choices that will ensure a lifetime of benefit and pleasure.

Invitation to my Facebook Page and Website

In the medical world information is continually being updated. I invite you to remain informed about advances in managing lymphedema by joining my Facebook group **Cooling for Lymphedema** where you can also ask questions or share experiences with the community.

And please visit my website at www.soflbreastrehab.org.

Conclusion

The use of cold therapy in treating inflammation and swelling may not be a new idea in rehabilitation, but its use in the clinical management of lymphedema represents a new use of a trusted ally. Having had the opportunity to treat acute cases of lymphedema in the oncologist's office made me aware that the application of topical skin cooling at the earliest expression of swelling, something which is not currently done as a standard of care, can potentially derail the progression of lymphedema to a chronic condition. My subsequent clinical observations and research findings revealed that cooling therapy has utility in resolving the underlying low-grade inflammation cause to the progressive development of lymphedema. This has opened my eyes to the need for an expanded definition of this condition. One that identifies the inflammation inherent in local post-surgical swelling and treats lingering inflammation more aggressively. A definition that will inspire clinicians to investigate new treatment options possibly including anti-inflammatory medical management options previously unforeseen. A definition that will help us better understand why lymphedema develops in some and not in others by learning about the role of the cumulative impact of chronic low-grade inflammatory processes on human health. Local swelling found postoperatively in delicate human tissue such as breast tissue is not commonly treated by topical skin cooling, presumably because up until now the utility of this modality in managing lymphedema had not yet been studied, and because delicate areas of the human body where sensation has been disrupted or altered by cancer related surgical and medical treatments require a more moderate approach to cooling therapy to prevent discomfort and further injury.

Those who oppose the use of cryotherapy have proven concerns about protecting delicate microvascular tissue from ischemia and permanent damage. The effectiveness of cancer therapies and the delivery of chemo therapy agents to cancer cells and tumors, depend on an intact and responsive microvasculature complex. Clearly preserving microvascular tissue is of great significance. We can learn to modify the application of cooling therapy, thereby deriving the anti-inflammatory benefits without placing sensitive tissue at risk. This draws attention to the discussion that dosing of cryotherapy is not yet common practice. More often than not, cooling therapy is randomly applied, without sufficient regard to the size of the area being treated and the depth of and length of time the cold temperature is allowed to penetrate into the tissue. Perhaps new technology can help to focus and target the practice of therapeutic cryotherapy and alleviate the concerns of overdosing and tissue damage.

Topical skin cooling positively impacts local as well as non-local lymphedema defined in this book for the first time, to distinguish between two distinct types of swelling the lymphedema specialist must be informed about and address.

Local swelling naturally occurs at the surgical site or after trauma. The edema consists of a mix of lymph and blood and extends through the layers incised by the surgical knife. Commonly we will see reparative fibrosis being formed as incisions are healed. Non-local swelling defines the accumulated lymph fluid present in the superficial lymphatics close to the outer layer of the dermis, the result of a breakdown in the system, that backs up through the vessels becoming stagnant in the interstitium and causing tissue distention and fibrosis. In this case fibrosis can be said to be reactive as it results in an excess deposit of extracellular matrix impeding function.

The main reason for making the distinction between local and non-local swelling is to clarify how delays in the resolve of local swelling, also referred to as temporary swelling postoperatively, can exacerbate the development of non-local lymphedema. When the resolution of temporary swelling is delayed and the inflammatory process appears to linger, such as seen in slow healing wounds or infections, tissue congestion occurs and reactive fibrosis is likely to develop, building on the reparative fibrous tissue already in place causing the scar to become more rigid. These processes impede lymphatic rerouting that is key to return of lymphatic function and explain why post-surgical infections are a known risk factor for developing secondary lymphedema. The use of post-surgical cooling therapy applied within the safe temperature range outlined in this book, supports local healing of tissue by resolving local swelling, discouraging lingering inflammation and preventing the deposit of excessive scar tissue associated with fibrosis. In addition, by decreasing the temperature in the tissue even though only slightly with the moderate temperatures defined, the risk of complications such as non-healing wounds and infections is theoretically also decreased as bacterial growth is impeded.

In non-local lymphedema, when the lymphatic fluid has backed up into the space around the cells, resulting in tissue congestion and fibrosis, cooling therapy effectively decreases tissue pressure, presumably by contraction of the arterioles and by decreasing venous intravascular pressure. Cooling also disburses trapped body heat, and in fact likely decreases the internal temperature of the superficial lymphatics. The full impact of moderate cooling on the superficial lymphatics is not yet known, although it would seem significant to the recovery of the contractile function of the all-important smooth muscle fibers that reside in the cell walls of the lymphangions if inflammation impeding the contractile function was reduced and the recovery of the involuntary lymphatic pump was supported before a total failure occurred. As tissue pressure decreases with cooling and pressure on nerve endings becomes less, clinically a rapid decrease in pain sensation was noted, often within the first cooling session, making moderate cryotherapy an effective and natural analgesic for nerve compression pain seen in lymphedema. In general the addition of cooling therapy was found to impact both local and non-local swelling positively and resulted in a faster return to functional mobility and the achievement of established therapy goals.

Scientific studies are evaluating the significance of the increased presence of macrophages, traditional markers of the inflammatory process, in areas of fibrosis related to lymphedema. Though results are still inconclusive, the question is already being raised just how much of lymphedema as we know its expression today is caused by a low-grade progressive inflammatory process? A process that we could potentially retard or reverse before permanent damage is done to the lymphatic system? Even more recent scientific information is allowing us to penetrate further into the intimate operations of the lymphatic system. The role of the Rho kinase pathway is of therapeutic interest as the contractile function of the lymphatic pump may well be found to be influenced by moderate cooling or by novel pharmaceuticals. The now proven ability of the lymphatic system to move molecules transcellular also gives us new appreciation for the obvious intelligence and resiliency of this system.

Based on current and ongoing clinical and scientific research, the therapeutic use of topical skin cooling in the clinical management of lymphedema has found new use as a viable treatment option for preventing and treating lymphedema. The novel use of cryotherapy for treating swelling associated with lymphedema already rests on the shoulders of this modality as a proven ally in rehabilitation. Clearly, a more moderate application of cooling is indicated given the proximity of the superficial lymphatics to the surface of the skin and the often sensitive areas of the human body involved. It would be prudent and kind for lymphedema medical practitioners to begin offering topical skin cooling treatment as a component of standard care in both local swelling immediately postoperatively, and in expressions of non-local or chronic lymphedema. Especially in the area of post-operative local swelling related to cancer surgeries, an area we have never before offered our best rehabilitation efforts, there appears to be a window to impact the development of chronic lymphedema. When cooling is applied within the safe temperature range described, the impact of low-grade inflammation on the lymphatic system is reduced and theoretically, the risk for developing chronic lymphedema will have been altered. Though it remains a topic for scientific debate and clinical monitoring, there is no reason to believe that providing preventative cryotherapy care within a moderate temperature range interferes with the body's natural reparative inflammatory response.

Topical skin cooling offers a new and much needed approach in the management of lymphedema. And though this book primarily discussed secondary lymphedema related to the breast and arm, the application of cooling holds promise for lymphedema resulting from other forms of cancer and other classifications of lymphedema. Having traveled in countries not so fortunate to have access to the high standards of lymphedema care customary in many developed countries, cooling therapy a treatment method that is available around the world where ever refrigeration is an option, has the potential to bring much needed relief to many who suffer. Topical skin cooling enhances the current offerings available for the management of this chronic condition by adding a solution that directly impacts the treatment of inflammation and expands the possibility for success. My vision is that the expression of lymphedema as we have come to accept it in the early 21st century, will be altered, as we continue to advance our knowledge and make new treatment options available. It is a journey well worth undertaking that will require the creative ideas and talents of the entire lymphedema community.

Jean Yzer is available for consultations and speaking engagements. For further information please visit www.soflbreastrehab.org.

Notes

CHAPTER 1

1. ACOLS – Academy of Lymphatic Studies
2. The American Physical Therapy Association Guide to Physical Therapy practice sections 6H Impaired Circulation and Anthropometric Dimensions Associated with Lymphatic System Disorders and 7H Primary Prevention/Risk reduction for Integumentary Disorders
3. The Lymphology Association of North America Position Paper on Lymphedema Risk Reduction Practices.

CHAPTER 2

4. Mayrovitz, HM, and Yzer, J, Local Skin Cooling as an Aid to the Management of Patients with Breast Cancer-Related Lymphedema and Fibrosis of the Arm or Breast, Lymphology 50(2017)56-66.
5. Zuther, Joachim, Lymphedema Management – The Comprehensive Guide for Practitioners, Thieme, Original publication December 2004
6. Triacca et al., Transcellular Pathways in Lymphatic Endothelial Cells Regulate Changes in Solute Transport by Fluid Stress. Circulation Research 2017;120:1440-1452. DOI:10.1161/CIRCRESAHA.116.309828.
7. Osiecki, H., The role of chronic inflammation in cardiovascular disease and its regulation by nutrients. Altern Med Rev. 2004 Mar;9(1):32-53.

CHAPTER 3

8. Block, Jon E., Cold and compression in the management of musculoskeletal injuries and orthopedic operative procedures: a narrative review, Open Access J Sports

Med. 2010; 1: 105-113. Published online 2010 Jul 7.
PMCID: PMC3781860

9. Weiss, JM, Treatment of leg edema and wounds in a pa-
    tient with severe musculoskeletal injuries, Phys Ther
    1998 Oct; 78(10):1104-13

10. Block, Jon E., Cold and compression in the management
    of musculoskeletal injuries and orthopedic operative
    procedures: a narrative review, Open Access J Sports
    Med. 2010; 1: 105-113. Published online 2010 Jul 7.
    PMCID: PMC3781860.

                        CHAPTER 4

11. Rakoff-Nahoum, S – Why Cancer and Inflammation?
    The Yale Journal of Biology and Medicine. 2006 Dec;
    79(3-4):123-130. Published online 2007 Oct.

12. Hutchison, Nancy A. MD, CLT-LANA Prophylactic An-
    tibiotics are an Important Adjunct to Decongestive
    Therapy for Recurrent Cellulitis in Lymphedema,
    NLNLymphlink Vol. 23 No. 3

13. Swapna Ghanta, Daniel A. Cuzzone, Jeremy S. Torrisi,
    Nicholas J. Albano, Walter J. Joseph, Ira L. Savetsky, Ja-
    son C. Gardenier, David Chang, Jamie C. Zampell, Ba-
    bak J. Mehrara Regulation of inflammation and fibrosis
    by macrophages in lymphedema American Journal of
    Physiology - Heart and Circulatory Physiology Pub-
    lished 1 May 2015 **Vol. 308 no.** 9, H1065-H1077 **DOI:**
    10.1152/ajpheart.00598.2014

14. C.E. Markhus, T.V. Karlsen, M. Wagner, Ø.S. Svendsen,
    O. Tenstad, K. Alitalo, H. Wiig Increased Interstitial
    Protein Because of Impaired Lymph Drainage Does Not
    Induce Fibrosis and Inflammation in Lymphedema. Ar-
    terioscler Thromb Vasc Biol is available at
    http://atvb.ahajournals.org.
    DOI: 10.1161/ATVBAHA.112.300384

                        CHAPTER 5

15. Christmas KM, Patik JC, Khoshnevis S, Diller KR, Brothers RM, Sustained cutaneous vasoconstriction during and following cryotherapy treatment: Role of Oxidative stress and Rho Kinase. Microvascular Res. 2016 Jul;106:96-100. Doi: 10.1016/j.mvr.2016.04.005.

16. Yao, L et al., The Role of RhoA/Rho kinase pathway in endothelial dysfunction. J Cardiovascular Disease Res. 2010 Oct-Dec; 1(4): 165-170 doi: 10.4103/0975-3583.74258

17. Hosaka H, Mizuno R, Ohhashi T, Rho-Rho kinase pathway is involved in the regulation of myogenic tone and pump activity in isolated lymph vessels. Am J Physiol Heart Circ Physiol 248: H2015-H2025, 2003;10.1152/ajpheart.00763.2002.

18. Mayrovitz, HM, and Yzer, J, Local Skin Cooling as an Aid to the Management of Patients with Breast Cancer-Related Lymphedema and Fibrosis of the Arm or Breast, Lymphology 50(2017)56-66.

19. Khoshnevis S, Craik NK, Matthew Brothers R, Diller KR, Cryotherapy-Induced Persistent Vasoconstriction After Cutaneous Cooling: Hysteresis Between Skin Temperature and Blood Perfusion, J Biomech Eng. 2016 Mar; 138(3):4032126. doi: 10.1115/1.4032126.

CHAPTER 7

20. Simmons, Holly, Preoperative Lymphedema Education for Breast Cancer Patients, Nursing and Health 3(3): 69-83, 2015 http://www.hrpub.org DOI: 10.13189/nh.2015.030303

CHAPTER 8

21. Burbach, JP, What are neuropeptides?, Methods Mol Biol. 2011;789:1-36. doi: 10.1007/978-1-61779-310-3_1.

22. Pert, Candace, Author of Molecules of Emotion: The Science Behind Mind-Body Medicine www.candacepert.com.

CHAPTER 9

23. NLN, National Lymphedema Network, www.lymphnet.org

24. Rehana L. Ahmed, William Thomas, Douglas Yee, Kathryn H. Schmitz, Randomized Controlled Trial of Weight Training and Lymphedema in Breast Cancer Survivors, DOI: 10.1200/JCO.2005.03.6749 Journal of Clinical Oncology 24, no. 18 (June 2006) 2765-2772.

25. Donald C. McKenzie, Andrea L. Kalda, Effect of Upper Extremity Exercise on Secondary Lymphedema in Breast Cancer Patients: A Pilot Study, DOI: 10.1200/JCO.2003.04.069 Journal of Clinical Oncology 21, no. 3 (February 2003) 463-466.

ABOUT THE AUTHOR

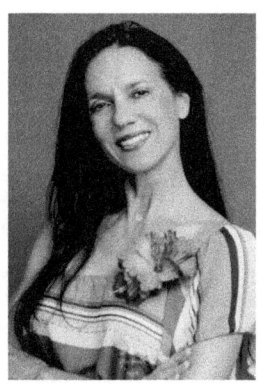

Jean A. Yzer has dedicated her professional life as a Physical Therapist to helping others on their journey from illness back to health. As a certified lymphedema therapist she had the intuitive knowing to make a seemingly unruly side-effect of cancer related treatments known as lymphedema become more manageable.

At her clinic *Total Lymphedema Care* in Pembroke Pines, Florida, Jean discovered that topical skin cooling has a therapeutic effect in the treatment of lymphedema. Her clinical judgment supports an emerging theory that chronic lymphedema must also be understood as a progressive inflammatory process, not just as the mechanical consequence of trauma it is more popularly understood to be. Jean co-authored a quantitative scientific study on the topic and demonstrated a reduction in the common symptoms of lymphedema when topical skin cooling was applied within a moderate temperature range determined to be safe for human tissue. She now leads the way in her profession instructing health professionals and patients alike in the use of topical skin cooling for the prevention and management of lymphedema. Jean is also the founder of The South Florida Breast Cancer Rehab Center, a non-profit organization whose mission is to advance the treatment of lymphedema.

Jean Yzer is available for consultations and speaking engagements. For further information please visit www.soflbreastrehab.org.

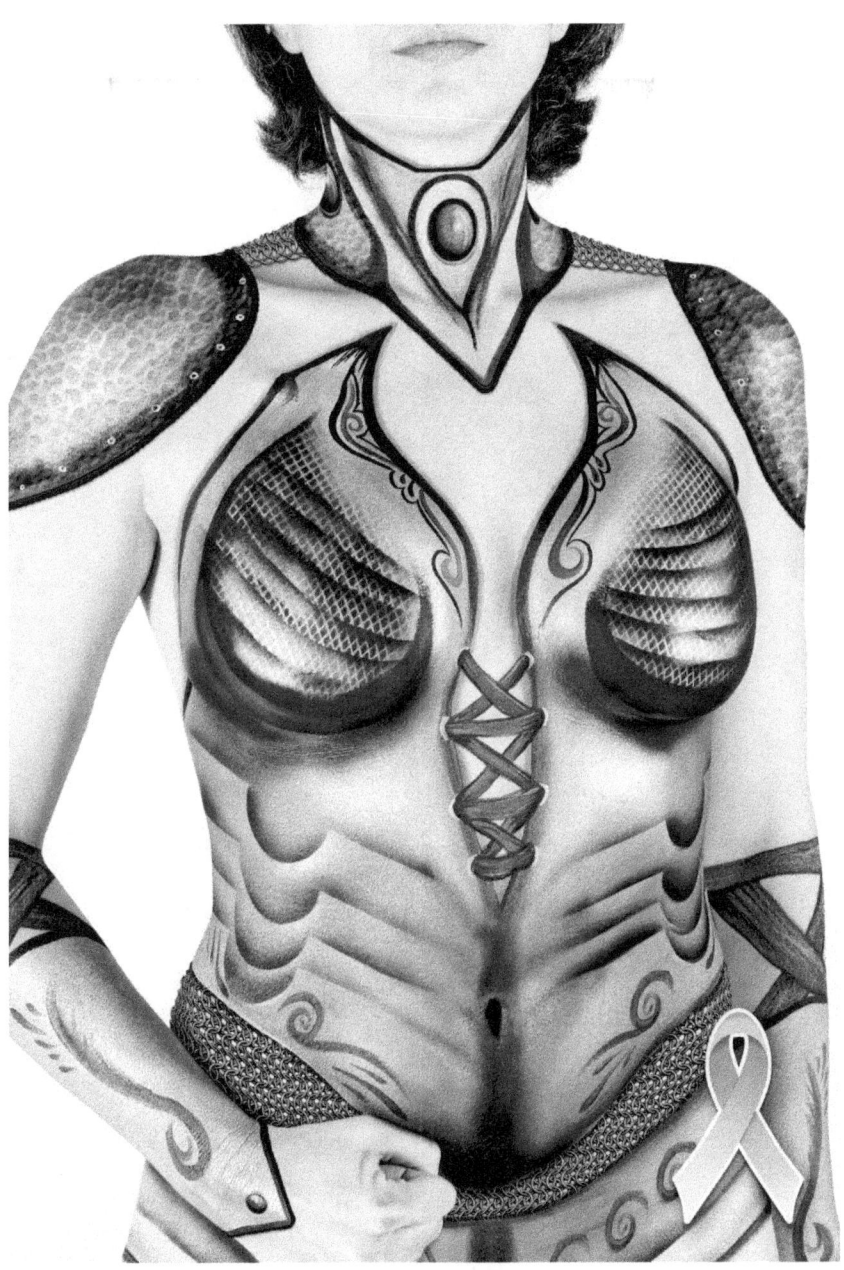

Warrior

www.ingramcontent.com/pod-product-compliance
Lightning Source LLC
Chambersburg PA
CBHW070138210526
45170CB00014B/1539